How to

More Energy

Guide to Naturally Increasing Your Physical and Mental Energy So You Can Accomplish Everything That Has to Get Done to Achieve Your Goals

By Jim Russlan

Contents

Thank you for buying this book and I hope that you will find it useful. If you will want to share your thoughts on this book, you can do so by leaving a review on the Amazon page, it helps me out a lot.

Introduction

Everybody struggles with exhaustion and fatigue in their lives for several reasons. Whether it's due to the fact that they work too much or do not get ample sleep during the night, or since they have a great deal of psychological baggage that drains their energy, or they eat an unhealthy diet plan.

For too long, we have been in a society that has actually trained us to look outside ourselves for the responses and expend our valuable energy generating things externally.

This sort of results-focused attitude induces us to disregard our inner strength, which leads to us being chronically tired and without energy.

Something that everybody requires to survive the daily grind is energy. Without it, we simply can't do what we need to do. The most substantial distinction between individuals who know what they desire and individuals who do not is energy. Every little thing that we do expends energy.

We use up energy each time we do, think, or express ourselves. Typically, we link the term energy with the physical version. Nevertheless, the reality is that energy is additionally utilized for other elements of day-to-day living.

Both emotional and mental energy are utilized daily, and so as to keep yourself effective and operational, you need to keep all 3 elements invigorated.

Regrettably, energy is not something that you can hold onto permanently. With each and every single action that you take, you use up energy. Every step that you take and every second you think cost you energy, and there is going to come a time when your energy is going to end up being diminished, and you'll end up being too tired to do anything.

If you do not look after yourself, there is going to come a time when you can't go on physically, emotionally, or mentally. You'll have pushed yourself to the limit. This is going to lead to what is called burnout.

Burnout can have a disastrous impact on your effectiveness, restricting the number of activities you can finish in a day, and the quality of those activities, and you will not have the ability to deal with your commitments.

Chapter 1—What is Fatigue

Prior to conquering your fatigue, you initially have to comprehend what fatigue is about. Fatigue is typically described as exhaustion or lethargy, and it is the sensation of weakness and low energy, both physically and psychologically.

You can experience short-term fatigue, which is an outcome of working too much or not getting ample rest. This type of fatigue could be quickly conquered. There is additionally chronic or medical fatigue, which is more long-lasting and needs more severe treatment.

According to the research, 10 percent of the world population experiences fatigue at any time, with women being impacted by fatigue more than guys. The majority of cases of fatigue have underlying psychological causes and 1 out of 5 individuals who suffer from fatigue in the US say that it impacts their regular functioning and every day lives.

Kinds Of Fatigue

There are 2 sorts of fatigue that you can experience, mental and physical fatigue. Physical fatigue is when you have a difficult time doing the important things that you typically do, like holding grocery bags or climbing up stairs. Physical exhaustion is simply not having ample physical strength to finish day-to-day activities.

Mental fatigue, conversely, is when you find it tough to focus on things. In extreme cases, you might discover even the act of getting out of bed to be excessive work.

You might feel exhausted all the time and might additionally struggle with a lower level of awareness, which could be exceptionally harmful, particularly when driving or running heavy machinery. If you experience mental fatigue, you might be mistaken for being intoxicated or drunk.

Weakness

Oftentimes, when describing fatigue, the words weakness and drowsiness are utilized to explain the condition. When the term weakness is utilized, it describes a scenario where your muscles simply do not have ample strength to finish even the rudimentary of physical activities.

When you experience weakness as a sign of fatigue, you frequently have to administer additional effort simply to move your legs, arms and other body parts. This is typically an outcome of overexerting yourself eventually, like when running a marathon or hiking the whole day.

Your body is going to feel weak and exhausted, and you'll experience some pains and aches. Thankfully, with ample rest, these signs are going to vanish after a number of days.

Drowsiness

Drowsiness, additionally referred to as somnolence, is when you feel sleepy even in the middle of an activity. This could be an outcome of not getting ample sleep, which is needed for you to feel invigorated and more unwinded.

What Causes Fatigue

To conquer fatigue, you need to know the source behind it. If you can remove the source from your life, you can completely eliminate fatigue from your life. The sources of fatigue could be divided into 3 primary groups: psychological, medical, and lifestyle.

Lifestyle Aspects

If you are experiencing fatigue, you might have to look thoroughly at your lifestyle. Consuming an excessive amount of caffeinated drinks or alcohol, having bad eating habits, substantial physical work, and not having the appropriate quantity of sleep can all add to fatigue in your life. To get rid of fatigue from your life, you'll need to think about changing your lifestyle.

Psychological Aspects

Your fatigue might additionally be an outcome of typical mental health problems. If you struggle with depression, anxiety, stress, or are handling grief; you can find your energy drained. These typical mental health problems can make you feel exhausted and lethargic.

Medical Aspects

In several circumstances, a medical condition can leave you feeling tired. In case you are experiencing persistent fatigue, it is necessary to speak with your physician to identify if you are experiencing a medical condition that is leading to chronic fatigue. Here are a few of the typical medical conditions that can lead to persistent fatigue.

- Depression is going to make you feel empty and sad, and it is going to additionally drain you of energy. It can induce you to lose sleep, which is going to lead to more fatigue. The initial step to remedying this problem is to look for expert assistance to attend to the issue.

- Diabetes is the body's failure to generate any or ample insulin to preserve good sugar levels. While Type 2 diabetes could be managed with working out and dieting, Type 1 is going to need medical intervention to keep it under control. Having unsteady blood sugar levels can cause fatigue and fatigue and can result in long-lasting harm to your body.

- Chronic Fatigue Syndrome can make you feel particularly disabling fatigue that is going to last for months. Causes could be mental, physical, or dietary. Nevertheless, there is no particular test that can detect chronic fatigue syndrome.

- Sleep Apnea is a condition that leads to periodic stopping and starting of your breathing while you sleep. This pattern is going to induce an absence of oxygen and an absence of sleep, leaving you feeling more worn out after sleeping than you did previously.

- Toxic Exposure can leave you feeling tired and empty. Chemical solvents, chlorine, dust, and other toxins and contaminants can lead to chronic fatigue, and they can additionally induce long-lasting harm to your body.

- Persistent inflammation is among the most typical reasons behind fatigue and could be brought on by inappropriate diet plan, stress, injury, and numerous other things. It is necessary to figure out the particular cause and get the appropriate treatment since, in addition to inducing fatigue, chronic inflammation can additionally cause long-lasting harm to skin, joints, and other organs.

- Nutritional Shortages are among the largest reasons behind fatigue and tiredness. When you are pushed to the limits mentally and physically, getting the appropriate fuel in your body is exceptionally crucial. A correct, well-balanced diet plan of fresh vegetables and fruit, grains, and lean meat is important for removing fatigue from your life.

To eliminate tiredness and fatigue, you need to determine the root causes of your condition.

Signs of Fatigue

The primary indication of fatigue is tiredness and exhaustion, particularly after finishing an exhausting physical activity or psychological exercise. While you might rest after the activity, your body and mind might still feel tired. Here are a few of the other signs of fatigue that you need to understand if you wish to find out how to conquer it.

Physical Signs

The physical signs of fatigue consist of aching muscles, abdominal pain, lightheadedness, bloating, headache, vision issues, and painful lymph nodes. In case you experience any of these signs for more than 2 weeks, it is necessary to speak to your physician to count out any typical conditions that can result in chronic fatigue.

If you are dealing with chronic fatigue, you might experience bad concentration, apathy, or an absence of motivation. You might additionally experience grumpiness, indecisiveness, hallucinations, frustration, memory problems, anorexia nervosa, sluggish reflexes and reactions to stimuli, bad judgment, and sleepiness.

By understanding these signs, you can determine if you are struggling with chronic fatigue or if you are simply tired and in requirement of a good night's sleep. Understanding the signs can assist you in discovering the appropriate remedy so you can eliminate your fatigue and improve your energy.

Chapter 2-- Eating Habits and Diet

Among the leading reasons for chronic fatigue is a bad diet plan. If you consume the incorrect foods frequently, you can start to feel exhausted and extremely tired. In order to get rid of tiredness and improve your energy levels, you have to stay clear of those foods that make you feel heavy and tired.

Which Foods Should You Eat

When you feel worn out, and your energy begins to subside, you might be lured to grab the sweet bar you have in your desk drawer. While it is going to offer you an instantaneous increase in energy, after about an hour, you'll be right back where you began. Rather than grabbing foods that are high in sugar, you have to consume foods that are high in protein and that have complex carbs.

Foods which contain complex carbs and are high in protein aid to boost your blood sugar levels and keep them at the appropriate level, offering your body the energy for a more prolonged duration. Complex carbs are additionally absorbed slower than simple carbohydrates, leading to you feeling fuller for longer.

During the day, you ought to attempt to take in whole grain items such as whole-grain crackers or whole-wheat bread. Include some low-fat cheese or peanut butter and another source of protein to keep you invigorated during the day.

Magnesium

So as to break down the glucose in your blood and convert it into energy, you have to take in Magnesium. Magnesium converts glucose into energy, and it is essential for the other 300 biochemical procedures that happen in your body.

When magnesium levels get too low, your energy level drops considerably, due to the fact that your glucose isn't being converted into energy correctly. Research studies have actually demonstrated that individuals who have magnesium shortages are most likely to tire quickly after doing physical activities.

Having low levels of magnesium can lead to quickly feeling out of breath and having a faster heart rate. This is an indicator that your body is working harder, which can rapidly zap your energy and make you feel tired.

It is essential that you get the advised quantity of magnesium in your diet plan if you wish to remove tiredness. Some outstanding sources of magnesium consist of fish, almonds, whole grains, cashews, and hazelnuts.

Eat Little Treats In Between Meals

It is far better to consume little meals with treats in between, instead of eating less regularly and overindulging during every meal. This is what is called power snacking.

By eating little treats in between meals, you keep your blood glucose up and your energy levels high. You can snack on fruits, yogurt, beef jerky, cheese, and nuts to stop you from getting too hungry in between meals.

Overindulging isn't great due to the fact that it can make you feel heavy and bloated, which can lead to feeling too lazy to move. To prevent overindulging, you might wish to think about placing your food on a tinier plate to offer the impression that your dish is full enough.

Drink A Lot Of Water

Drinking ample water daily enhances your general health and wellness, and it can assist you to stay clear of feeling weak and tired. Water keeps your body hydrated at all times, which can assist in protecting against fatigue. To maximize the power of water, you ought to take in a minimum of 8 cups of water every day. Otherwise, you'll feel lethargic for the whole day.

Incorporate Soluble Fiber in Your Diet

Soluble fiber assists your body to take in sugars more gradually, which is essential for you to get a more lasting level of energy. When your body soaks up sugar too rapidly, it can result in an abrupt crash right after the sugar high. You can obtain soluble fiber from eating fruits, nuts, veggies, oats, whole grains, and beans.

Utilize Caffeine in Small Amounts

Stimulants such as soda, coffee, and nicotine can rapidly tire your adrenaline glands, making you feel exhausted for prolonged time periods. Coffee and other caffeinated items can provide you with the fast energy increase that you require, however, it can end up being detrimental if you end up being dependent on it. If you wish to get rid of fatigue, then you need to stop taking in things that provide you with a fast energy increase.

Consume Foods that Detoxify You

In case you have a tendency to feel worn out and tired constantly, there are a number of foods that you can consume to cleanse your mind and body.

Eating broccoli and cabbage is going to assist in cleaning damaging toxic substances from your liver, and are both abundant in anti-oxidants. Consuming beets can assist in cleaning your body while getting rid of free radicals. Other foods that can assist in cleansing your body are asparagus, garlic, lemongrass, wheatgrass, green tea, and avocados.

Meal Timing

Correctly timing your meals can have an extensive impact on your energy and metabolism. Eating too little or too much can make you feel sluggish and can interrupt blood glucose levels, leading to chronic fatigue. Timing your meals is going to guarantee that you are going to have ample energy to survive the day and accomplish your activities without feeling tired later.

We have all heard that "breakfast is the most important meal of the day," and for an excellent reason. Breakfast is the initial meal of the day and serves as the fuel that you require to keep going. Consuming a dietary breakfast makes you more effective and lively in the early morning and assists to keep you sustained during the morning.

In case you have a rewarding meal in the early morning, you can get away with consuming a lighter lunch and supper. Overindulging in the nights and afternoons can make you feel slow and really decrease the energy you need to get you through the remainder of the day.

Maintaining a healthy diet plan and taking in the appropriate types of foods at the correct times during the day can assist you to remove fatigue and improve your energy levels. Following the above suggestions is going to keep your energy levels high during the day and enable you to achieve more in your day.

Chapter 3—How to Chance the Lifestyle

Another reason for fatigue could be having a substandard lifestyle. The bad sort of lifestyle is going to induce exhaustion and fatigue, in addition to a variety of other health issues in your life.

You might not know it; however, the important things that you do daily might be adding to your consistent tiredness and fatigue. To work toward lastly eliminating fatigue, you have to understand how to tweak your lifestyle to keep your energy levels high.

Exercise Enough

Among the principles of energy management is discovering how to look after your body. Looking after it well enables you to keep going for prolonged durations of time. Among the necessary elements of looking after your body is working out.

You might believe that attempting to work out when you are tired is detrimental. Nevertheless, working out is incredibly helpful in combating fatigue. Exercise assists in enhancing your muscle strength and endurance and that makes you feel less worn out as time passes.

It additionally aids to disperse the oxygen and nutrients to your cells, which enable your body to work more effectively. When your body works more effectively, you do not feel as worn out when you take part in physical activity due to the fact that your body does not need to work double-time.

Why You Should Be Working Out

- It keeps your body in exceptional condition, which is very important when it comes to keeping your energy levels up. When you get enough exercise, you cultivate physical endurance. This is particularly true when you take part in cardio. By simply getting into shape, you can have more energy to endure the daily grind.

- It's an outlet for stress release. Stress can make you fed up physically, and it can induce you to end up being fed up both mentally and emotionally. Having an outlet to discharge tension is essential for keeping you strong. There are numerous methods through which you can discharge tension, however, among the very best methods is physical exercise.

- It can assist you in shaping your body. As your muscles end up being more defined, your body works more effectively.

- It can alleviate you of the impacts of chronic fatigue. Fatigue can have a destructive effect on your life. Among the very best methods to decrease the effect of fatigue is working out frequently. Routine exercise enhances your joints and muscles that might be worn out due to work.

There are lots of manners in which you can boost your levels of physical activity to assist with boosting your energy. You can head to the gym, you can go out for a jog, or you can take part in a sport on the weekends. Here are some other types of exercise to get rid of exhaustion.

Yoga

Practicing yoga is going to assist with boosting your energy, and it is additionally exceptional for restoring your balance. Practicing yoga regularly can assist you in handling stress, and it can lessen the signs of depression. It is understood to assist with enhancing versatility, along with boosting metabolic rate while increasing your cardiovascular health.

Walking or Running

Running and walking are excellent methods to get your heart pumping and your body going. In addition to boosting your energy levels, walking or running can assist in enhancing your general health and helping with the avoidance of numerous illnesses.

Having a walking or running routine can assist in easing stress, which can rapidly zap your energy levels. These types of workouts can additionally lessen signs of depression. In addition to providing you with an instantaneous increase in energy, it can additionally assist in clearing your mind.

Tai Chi

Tai Chi is among the most prominent sorts of exercises in the East. Tai Chi can boost your vigor and assist you in fighting stress. It can additionally enhance your cognitive function while successfully raising your energy levels. It can additionally enhance your quality of sleep, which is huge when it pertains to restoring your energy and vigor.

Dancing

Dancing is among the most pleasurable types of exercise. It can assist you in fighting stress while toning your muscles. Taking part in an arranged dance lesson or simply going out for an enjoyable night of dancing on a Friday night can make you feel happy, which could be very helpful when you are combating fatigue.

You do not need to dedicate yourself to intense workouts to take advantage of exercising. Something as easy as tweaking your typical inactive regimen may do a lot for your energy and total health. Think about taking the stairs instead of getting the elevator, or parking farther away from the shop when out shopping.

You can additionally attempt brand-new pastimes that consist of exercising, such as playing sports, cycling, or hiking. These basic and enjoyable activities can assist in making your body stronger and reducing fatigue. As you start to end up being more physically active, you are going to observe a considerable boost in your energy, making finishing your day-to-day activities a lot easier.

Get Enough Sleep

Another reason you might be experiencing fatigue and exhaustion is that you aren't getting ample rest and recuperative sleep. If you attempt to do a lot of activities at one time, you'll wind up mentally and physically worn out, which can rapidly cause fatigue. This is why it is so crucial to provide your mind and body a break and time to recuperate after doing something that is especially strenuous or demanding.

Usually, many people need 8 hours of sleep every night. To guarantee that you get the sleep you require, it is vital to set a routine bedtime and get up at the same time each day to permit your body to get used to the regimen.

When you get adequate sleep during the night, you are going to naturally get up, without needing to depend on the alarm. It is far better for your physical and psychological health to get up by yourself, instead of depending on an alarm.

In case you aren't able to obtain 8 hours of sleep, you can offset the lost sleep hours by taking a nap throughout the day. This is going to enable you to catch up on sleep without interfering with your routine sleep patterns.

Another method to keep yourself from ending up being excessively fatigued is resting your mind and body after finishing activities. Make use of breaks at work carefully to end up being more effective and efficient. When you are doing household chores, make certain to pause so you can re-energize your body.

Eliminate Bad Habits and Vices

Your bad habits, such as drinking alcohol, smoking cigarettes, or consuming excessive caffeine and sugar, can substantially add to your fatigue. Alcohol has a sedative impact that leads to your body feeling heavy. You ought to stay clear of having an afternoon drink, particularly in case you still have plenty of activities to finish prior to calling it a day.

You might be in the routine of drinking alcohol after supper or prior to going to sleep due to the fact that you believe that it assists you to sleep much better. Nevertheless, alcohol stops your body and mind from entering into a deep sleep, leading to you not feeling rested and revitalized, even in case you obtain the suggested 8 hours of sleep during the night.

Smoking cigarettes can additionally zap your energy due to the fact that it stops you from obtaining a good night's sleep. Individuals who stopped smoking cigarettes have actually declared that their energy levels double, and often triple, after eliminating a bad habit. Smoking cigarettes can induce you to feel grouchy, moody, and irritable throughout the day, which can drain your energy. In case you wish to boost your energy and remove fatigue, you have to discover how to stop smoking cigarettes.

In addition to impacting your energy and inducing you to be more tired, alcohol intake and smoking cigarettes can have other negative impacts on your body that can substantially affect your health.

Participate in a Relaxing Hobby

Together with taking part in pastimes that need you to use up energy, such as dancing, hiking, or a range of sports, you ought to additionally take part in hobbies that are relaxing. Pastimes that promote relaxation are excellent for when you want to relax after a long day at work.

Instead of grabbing the television remote, you want to discover a relaxing activity such as reading or gardening. Regrettably, the TV needs your mind to keep on work, and that can boost your stress, even if you are simply resting on the sofa.

Taking part in unwinding activities such as woodworking or baking is going to unwind both your body and mind since they do not require you to overthink and are not physically laborious.

Meditation

Meditation is an effective tool that you can utilize to assist you in handling your stress, getting rid of tiredness, and enhancing the total quality of your life. It has actually additionally been demonstrated to enhance your cognitive function and boost your energy and vigor when practiced routinely.

When you practice meditation routinely, you are, in reality, training your body to unwind. When you rest, you reduced the levels of cortisol that your body is generating. Cortisol is called the stress hormone since it is discharged when you end up being stressed. High levels of cortisol in your blood are related to boosted blood pressure, stress, fatigue, and weight gain.

If you are a beginner when it comes to meditation, here's how to obtain the most benefits from every session.

- Sit or lie cozily. You might wish to buy an excellent cushion or meditation chair to guarantee that you are comfy during the whole session.

- Shut your eyes.

- Breathe naturally. Attempt to stay clear of attempting to manage your breathing. Simply breathe in and breathe out as you generally would.

- Start to concentrate your attention on your breath and how your body shifts with each exhalation and inhalation. Observe the motion of your body as you breathe. Observe your shoulders, chest, rib cage, and belly. Concentrate your attention on your breathing, avoiding attempting to manage its intensity or pace. In case you discover that your mind is straying, return your focus back to your breath.

Sustain your meditation for 2 to 3 minutes when you are first beginning. As soon as you discover that you can sustain your focus for 3 minutes, you can begin increasing the duration of every session. There are no genuine drawbacks to meditation and could be exceptionally unwinding and assist with alleviating signs of fatigue.

Listen to Unwinding Music

Current studies have actually demonstrated that listening to calming music can minimize anxiety, stress, and fatigue. It has actually likewise been demonstrated to assist you in getting a good night's sleep, efficiently lowering the impacts of sleeping disorders, which can assist you to battle fatigue further.

Music assists to relax us, unwind our muscles, minimize stress, reduce blood pressure, and enhance the heart rate. It works in the same manner as meditation. To assist in getting rid of stress and boosting your energy, attempt listening to calming music, in the mornings and prior to going to sleep during the night.

Chapter 4-- Organize Your Life

Something that can induce you to end up being tired are turmoil and mess in your life. If you wish to be devoid of exhaustion and fatigue, then you have to keep your home, work area, and life arranged. There are lots of things that you may do to produce a more orderly life.

Create Lists

Making a note of every little thing that you have to achieve and remember throughout the day makes it simpler for you to carry out your everyday activities. Attempting to bear in mind every little thing that you have to attain throughout the day can drain your energy. By producing lists, you remove the requirement to make an effort remembering and keeping in mind every little thing you need to do.

When you go grocery shopping, you have to create a list of the important things that you have to purchase so that you do not need to use up energy attempting to recall what you require. At the end of the day, develop a list of the activities that you have to do the following day.

Another list you ought to think about making is the list of your month-to-month costs so that you can plan your budget. You can create your lists in an organizer or a little note pad, or use one of the many organization apps for your smartphone. Whichever you pick, simply ensure you're producing your lists daily.

Make Due Dates and Schedules

Another manner in which you can arrange your life much better is by producing due dates and schedules for all the important things that you have to do. This can assist you to stay clear of squandering your time, which is going to offer you the time you require to rest and unwind and renew your energy. If you aren't able to handle your time efficiently, you'll just wind up attempting to complete every little thing in the nick of time, which can make you feel tired.

By developing due dates and schedules on your own, you understand what has to be done, and you can concentrate your effort on one activity at a time. It is essential to keep in mind to set practical schedules and due dates to stay clear of ending up being more exhausted and stressed out.

Don't Procrastinate

Falling under a habit of procrastination just makes your activities harder when it's time to finish them. Putting things off simply makes you more stressed out since you need to hurry things up to meet the due dates that you set. Procrastination is going to additionally induce you to generate low-grade outcomes.

If you start your activities at the earliest possible time, you can take more time to finish them without needing to complete them in a small quantity of time. Additionally, when you can complete an activity prior to its due date, it offers you much more time to kick back and unwind to restore your energy.

When you develop a schedule and set due dates, it is essential that you stay with it. To assist with getting rid of tiredness, you have to find out how to concentrate on finishing the activity at hand while avoiding interruptions, like social media, e-mail, or your phone.

Prioritize

While producing a schedule is a good idea, a long to-do-list can end up being frustrating. To avoid ending up being fatigued at the thought of finishing every little thing on your schedule, you have to find out how to prioritize. To assist you in prioritizing the activities that you have to carry out, have a look at your list and choose which tasks need to be finished that day and which ones could be moved to a different day.

For instance, if it's June and you included shopping for school materials on your list of things to accomplish, in addition to everything else that you have to accomplish, you might start to feel overloaded and too tired by the time you get to the end of your list.

To repair this, move the activity of shopping for school materials, and other things that you do not have to finish right now, to another day, offering you the time to finish the activities with the closest due date.

Declutter Your Work area

Another method to keep your life arranged is to declutter your work area. Doing away with clutter at your desk is going to aid you in being more effective throughout the day. Prior to leaving for the day, make it a point to clear off the surface of your desk, making certain to put every little thing back where it belongs. Do not leave folders and files piled on top of your desk.

Rather, designate a tray for all your outbound and inbound files. Put any materials that you do not require right away into a file cabinet. It is going to be a lot easier for you to work when every little thing is put in its appropriate spot, so you do not need to lose time looking for things you require.

If you wish to have a place to rest and unwind, then you'll need to declutter your home. A tidy and well-organized home is going to make it a lot easier for you to unwind your worn-out mind and body. Having a messy home is going to just result in you feeling more tired and stressed out, which could be a contributing aspect to your tiredness and fatigue. You need to do away with your home's clutter if you wish to work toward getting rid of fatigue from your life.

While it is going to take some effort and time upfront, decluttering your home now is going to be well worth it to get rid of fatigue from your life. Begin by going through your things and removing anything that you no longer require or have any use for, such as toys, old clothes, DVDs, or books.

You can either donate the things to charity or hold a garage sale. In case you discover things that are broken and that are irreparable, toss them out. At the end of the day, you just wish to have things at home that you still utilize. To keep your house clutter-free, you have to have a place to place every little thing. You ought to use drawers, shelves, and cabinets to lessen the clutter and make it simpler to locate what you are searching for. You additionally wish to restrict the number of things that you buy. Prior to purchasing anything, you have to ask yourself if it is something that you actually require.

Delegate

Another excellent method to stop yourself from ending up being fatigued is delegating activities. Comprehending that you do not need to do every little thing yourself could be very advantageous when it comes to lowering fatigue and boosting your energy. You can delegate activities both at work and in your private life. If you are a supervisor of a manager, discover how to delegate activities to your people properly. When you are at home, get the aid of your youngsters and other family members to finish chores. It is important to ensure that you additionally deal with your obligations without depending upon others to do every little thing for you.

The Power of No

To prevent tiredness, you have to discover what your constraints are both psychologically and physically. It is essential that you find out how to say 'no' if you do not believe that you can handle any more activities or obligations.

Improve Your Energy.

You do not need to work overtime whenever your employer asks you to, and you do not need to take part in every social engagement that turns up. You have to discover how to listen to your body and discover how to decline invites and demands nicely.

Chapter 5-- Avoid Stress.

If you wish to stay clear of tiredness, then you have to find out about the various stress management strategies that can assist you in handling your emotions. When stress is left unmanaged, it can rapidly drain you of all your energy.

Severe levels of stress could be dangerous if you do not make an effort to handle the stress right away. It can impact your cognitive function and energy levels, in addition to altering the general quality of your life. It is essential to find out how to reduce stress in your life if you wish to remove tiredness and improve your energy.

Do not Be So Tough on Yourself

The majority of the stress that we experience in our lives is self-induced. If you wish to fight stress and remove tiredness from your life, then you need to stay clear of being too tough on yourself.

Stay clear of burning the candle at both ends. Make an effort to unwind and recharge yourself and stay clear of working too hard and pressing yourself to the point of burnout.

Forget About Perfectionism

Many individuals continually opt for perfectionism. The issue with this is that you are continuously setting yourself up to fall short by setting impractical standards for yourself. Among the most effective methods by which you can handle anxiety and stress in your life is forgetting about perfectionism.

Nevertheless, you should constantly do your finest each time you concentrate on an activity. The vital part is acknowledging that your finest is good enough.

Do not Take Yourself Too Seriously

This life is complicated enough as it is, do not contribute to your stress by taking life and yourself too seriously. If you intend to live a delighted and worry-free life, you need to cultivate an excellent sense of humor.

It is crucial that you find out how to laugh at yourself. There is constantly something amusing in every circumstance that you find yourself in, even the hardest situations. Discovering humor in life is going to assist you to feel much better and is going to immediately boost your energy.

Speak with Somebody

Get the assistance of a specialist. Speaking to somebody about your life, both the bad and good parts of it can assist you in handling the stress and boosting the quantity of energy you have daily.

Talking with an expert can assist you in understanding that you aren't alone in your worries and issues. Speaking to somebody that you trust could be extremely restorative and assist you in finding out how to handle your stress much better.

Be Clear About Your Objectives

To stay clear of spreading yourself too thin, it is vital that you are clear about what you wish to accomplish. Begin setting clear goals in every part of your life, consisting of career, finances, personal development, relationships, and health. Understanding precisely what you have to do to accomplish your objectives is going to keep you from ending up being excessively tired and stressed.

Stop Attempting to Manage Every Little Thing

There will be things that show up in your life that you can't manage. If you wish to live a delighted, worry-free, and high energy life, then you have to concentrate your energy on those things in your life that you can manage, and you need to discover how to let go of the things that you can't manage.

Take Deep Breaths

When you are feeling stressed out or excessively fatigued, taking a couple of slow, deep breaths is going to assist you to unwind. Take a second to inhale as far as you can, and breathe out as much as you can. Do this 3-5 times, gradually, and you are going to feel the impacts on your fatigue and stress levels instantly.

Besides handling your stress, you have to find out how to manage your feelings if you wish to get rid of exhaustion to boost your energy. Harmful feelings, such as jealousy, anger, guilt, and resentment are going to drain your energy and boost your levels of fatigue, stress, anxiety, and lead to depression.

Damaging emotions can use up all your energy, and they can draw out all the positivity in your life. Knowing how to manage your emotions is going to minimize your tiredness and boost your energy.

Forgive Yourself

If you constantly feel guilty about things that you have done in the past, you are just going to boost your levels of stress and fatigue. You need to discover how to forgive yourself for your past mistakes and misgivings if you wish to live a life devoid of fatigue and stress.

When you find out how to forgive yourself, you are going to see an instant boost in your vigor and energy, along with better health.

Forgive Other People

Among the quickest methods to drain your energy and develop stress and anxiety in your life is to hold onto grudges. For you to boost your energy and vigor, you need to find out how to forgive those who have actually hurt you before.

Forgiving them does not imply that you are excusing their actions, and it does not imply that you need to invite them back into your life. Forgiveness just implies that you are prepared to let go of the past hurt and that you are ready to live the life that you should have.

Have Healthy Personal Boundaries

You might believe that you wish to please everybody around you. Nevertheless, attempting to please everybody all the time can end up being extremely discouraging and result in boosted levels of fatigue and stress. If you wish to enhance your emotions and boost your energy, you have to produce healthy personal boundaries.

Taking part in people-pleasing behavior frequently drains your energy since you wind up spreading yourself too thin. Keep in mind that it's alright to say no to demands that do not serve your best interests. Having healthy personal boundaries is among the most effective manners in which you can protect against stress in your life to get rid of fatigue.

You need to discover how to handle your emotions and stress if you wish to live a high energy life. If you discover that it's inconceivable to stay clear of some demanding scenarios, then it is in your best interest to handle these circumstances as gently and as objectively as you can.

Conclusion

When dealing with persistent fatigue, the first thing that you ought to do is count out any medical condition that you might have. If you do have one of the numerous medical conditions that add to persistent tiredness, the very best thing you may do is taking your physician's suggestions and abiding by any treatment plan they suggest.

If a medical condition has actually been ruled out as an explanation for your continuous fatigue, then it's most likely that your present way of life is adding to your exhaustion. The bright side is that it could be reversed so that you can have more energy.

Concentrating on changing your lifestyle and doing what you may in order to get rid of stress from your life is going to assist you in improving your energy and rebuilding your vigor, getting rid of fatigue completely.

While you most likely will not have the ability to significantly alter your whole way of life overnight, you can quickly focus on a handful of the more crucial things. Even the tiniest modifications in your way of life are going to assist in enhancing your energy.

To efficiently fight fatigue and boost your energy, you simply have to take things one day at a time and concentrate on being a much better version of yourself. Every small change that you make is going to have a substantial effect on your total health, vigor, and energy. You do not need to continue to live with fatigue and tiredness.

Making straightforward changes in your diet and everyday life can assist you to discover the energy you require to make it through your days. There is absolutely nothing like having the ability to live a complete and effective life with ample energy to make it through even the most difficult of activities.

I hope that you enjoyed reading through this book and that you have found it useful. If you want to share your thoughts on this book, you can do so by leaving a review on the Amazon page. Have a great rest of the day.

Printed in Great Britain
by Amazon